Summary

1. Introduction

Objective and philosophy of the book

Dear readers,

Welcome to this unique journey, where we will explore the physical and mental well-being world for those over 60. Our journey will share adapted physical exercises, nutritional advice, and a holistic vision of well-being that embraces body, mind, and spirit.

Our main objective is twofold. First, I want to equip you with knowledge and tools to nourish your body in a balanced way, considering the specific nutritional needs of this beautiful stage of life. Second, I will guide you through exercises, from stretching to Pilates and yoga practices, that you can do comfortably at home, regardless of whether you have equipment. These exercises have been selected and adapted to improve flexibility, physical strength, and mental and emotional well-being.

The philosophy guiding this book is that each of you is unique in your needs, abilities, and limitations. For this reason, every advice, exercise, and nutritional suggestion is designed to be flexible and adaptable to your conditions. I hope these pages become a source of inspiration and support for taking care of yourself lovingly and consciously.

This book promises sustainable change towards a healthier and more active lifestyle. I won't offer you quick fixes or fads but achievable and enjoyable practices that you can easily integrate into your daily life. And remember, every small step you take on this journey is a cause for celebration, a sign of progress toward a fuller, more satisfying life.

Thank you for embarking on this journey with me. I am excited to accompany you, sharing my knowledge, exercises, and nutritional advice to help you live daily with more energy, health, and happiness.

With love and dedication,

Giuseppe Di Mauro

How to use this book

This book was created as a guide and companion on your path to a healthier and more active life, especially for those in your 60s. Here are some tips on how to best use it:

1. **Read with an Open and Personalized Approach**: Each individual has unique needs and abilities. As you explore

the various chapters, consider how each suggestion fits your circumstances. Don't hesitate to modify the exercises or nutritional advice based on your needs and preferences.

2. **Start with the Section That Interests You Most**: Following the book in order is unnecessary. If you are particularly interested in nutrition or stretching exercises, start there. The important thing is that you feel comfortable and motivated.

3. **Set Realistic Goals**: As you work through this book, set short- and long-term goals for your health and well-being. Considering your current fitness level and health condition, these goals should be realistic and achievable.

4. **Create a Daily Routine**: Try to integrate the practices suggested in the book into your daily routine. Even a few minutes a day dedicated to exercise or meal planning can make a big difference.

5. **Use the Book as a Journal**: Consider keeping notes in the margins or a separate journal. Write down which exercises work best for you, which foods make you feel more energetic, and your progress over time.

6. **Listen to Your Body**: Listen to your body during exercises. If you feel pain or discomfort, stop. The golden rule is to proceed gradually and without force.

7. **Reread the Sections That Struck You**: Don't hesitate to return to chapters or sections that particularly struck or inspired you. Sometimes, rereading with a new perspective can offer additional insights.

8. **Share Your Experiences**: If you feel comfortable, share what you learn or your progress with friends or family. Sometimes, sharing your journey can provide additional motivation and support.

Remember, this book is more than just a guide; it is an invitation to care for yourself more consciously and joyfully. Every step you take, every new habit you integrate into your life, is a step towards better health and more happiness.

Have a good wellness journey.

2. Nutrition Fundamentals for Over 60s

Principles of a healthy diet for seniors

Maintaining a healthy and balanced diet is essential at any age, but it becomes even more crucial when you reach the age of 60. Here are some fundamental principles for a healthy diet for Seniors :

1. **Nutritional Balance**: Make sure your diet includes a good balance of macronutrients (proteins, carbohydrates, and fats) and various micronutrients (vitamins and minerals). This helps keep the body strong and prevent nutritional deficiencies.

2. **Quality Proteins**: Proteins are essential for preserving muscle mass, which tends to decrease with age. Include lean protein sources such as chicken, fish, legumes, eggs, and low-fat dairy products.

3. **Fiber for Digestion**: Fiber plays a vital role in digestion and maintaining intestinal health. Fruits, vegetables, whole grains, and legumes are excellent sources of fiber.

4. **Calcium and Vitamin D for Bones**: As we age, bones weaken, making calcium and vitamin D important. Foods such as fortified milk, yogurt, cheese, leafy green vegetables, and fatty fish can help.

5. **Adequate hydration**: Older people may not feel thirsty as intensely as they once did. Therefore, drinking water regularly during the day is essential for good hydration.

6. **Limit Sugars and Saturated Fats: Reducing your intake of added sugars and saturated fats can help prevent chronic diseases such as type** 2 diabetes and cardiovascular disease.

7. **Adequate Portions**: Your calorie needs may decrease as you age. It's essential to listen to your body and adjust your food portions to maintain a healthy body weight.

8. **Antioxidant-Rich Foods**: Antioxidant-rich foods like colorful fruits and vegetables can help fight inflammation and reduce the risk of chronic disease.

9. **Sodium Reduction**: Excessive sodium intake is associated with blood pressure problems. Limit salt and use herbs and spices to flavor your dishes.

10. **Regularity in Meals**: Eating at regular times helps keep energy and blood sugar levels stable.

Remember that these principles are general guidelines. Individual needs may vary, so it is always advisable to consult a health professional for specific advice. A well-balanced diet and regular physical activity can significantly affect your health and well-being.

Integration and hydration

An essential component of maintaining a healthy lifestyle, especially in old age, is understanding the importance of supplementation and hydration. Let's see together how to manage them best.

Integration

As you age, your body may have nutritional needs that can't always be met through diet alone. This is why integration can play a crucial role:

1. **Vitamins and Minerals**: As we age, the absorption of some nutrients may decrease. Supplements such as vitamin D, B12, calcium, and iron can be helpful, but it is essential to consult your doctor before starting any supplement regimen.

2. **Omega-3 fatty acids**: Omega-3 fatty acids, found in fish and some supplements, are known for their benefits on heart and brain health.

3. **Probiotics**: Maintaining good gut health is crucial. Probiotic supplements can help, especially if you have digestive problems.

4. **Personalized Integration**: Each individual has different needs. Discuss which supplements are best for you with your doctor, considering your overall health and any medications you take.

Hydration

Hydration is vital for all ages but even more critical for seniors. Here's how to make sure you drink enough:

1. **Water First**: Water should be your primary source of hydration. Always drink regularly throughout the day, even if you don't feel thirsty.

2. **Recognizing the Signs of Dehydration**: Dehydration in Seniors may not always be apparent. Tiredness, confusion, dry mouth, and dark urine are signs not to be underestimated.

3. **Water-rich foods**: Fruits and vegetables with high water content, such as watermelon, cucumbers, and tomatoes, can help with hydration.

4. **Avoid Dehydrating Drinks**: Limit consumption of coffee, tea, and alcohol, as they can contribute to dehydration.

5. **Create a Hydration Plan**: If you find it challenging to remember to drink, try establishing a hydration plan, such as drinking a glass of water with each meal and one between meals.

6. **Monitor Fluid Intake**: Follow your doctor's recommendations if you have medical conditions requiring fluid restriction, such as kidney or heart problems.

Remember, supplementation and adequate hydration are critical to your health and well-being. Take these aspects with the seriousness they deserve, always by your doctor's advice.

Take care of yourself with love and awareness.

Weight management in old age

Weight management in later life is crucial to maintaining a healthy and active lifestyle. Here are some tips on effectively managing your weight during these precious years.

1. **Balancing Calories and Physical Activity**: As you age, your body may require fewer calories due to a natural reduction in metabolism and physical activity. It is essential to balance caloric intake with physical activity. Light but regular exercise, such as walking, swimming, or yoga, can help you maintain a healthy weight.

2. **Nutritious and Balanced Nutrition**: Focus on nutrient-rich, low-calorie-density foods. This means choosing foods that provide lots of vitamins, minerals, and fiber but fewer calories. Fruits, vegetables, whole grains, and lean proteins should be the basis of your diet.

3. **Track Servings**: It's significantly more straightforward to consume more calories than you need if your eating habits don't change as your calorie needs decrease. Use smaller plates and control portion sizes to avoid overeating.

4. **Avoid Empty Foods and Unhealthy Snacks**: Limit your consumption of low-nutrient but high-calorie foods, such as sweets, processed snacks, and sugary drinks.

5. **Maintain Adequate Hydration**: Sometimes, the feeling of hunger can be a sign of dehydration. Make sure you drink water regularly throughout the day.

6. **Check** Your Weight Regularly: Monitoring your weight regularly can help you quickly recognize any changes and adjust your diet and exercise regimen accordingly.

7. **Consult Health Professionals**: If you have concerns about weight management, do not hesitate to consult your doctor or a nutritionist. They can provide personalized recommendations based on your health conditions, nutritional needs, and physical activity.

8. **Holistic Approach to Wellness**: Remember that weight management is not just about the numbers on the scale. It's also a matter of maintaining a balance between mind, body, and spirit. Do activities that make you happy,

socialize, and dedicate time to hobbies and interests that enrich your life.

Remember, weight is only one part of your journey to health and wellness. The main goal should always be to live a whole, active, and satisfying life.

Practical recipes and meal plans

Incorporating healthy recipes and practical meal plans into your daily routine can make a big difference on your path to wellness. Here are some ideas to help you get started.

Simple and nutritious recipes

1. **Fruit and Vegetable Smoothies**: Start your day with a nutritious smoothie. Combine fresh or frozen fruit, leafy greens, a pinch of ginger for digestion, and a protein source such as Greek yogurt or protein powder.

2. **Colorful Salads**: For a light lunch, try a salad with vegetables, some lean protein like chicken, tuna, or legumes, and a dressing made from olive oil and lemon. Add a handful of dried fruit for a touch of crunch.

3. **Soups and Stews**: Prepare soups and stews rich in vegetables, legumes, and lean meats. They are easy to

cook in large quantities and perfect for storing and reheating.

4. **Baked Fish with Vegetables**: Fish is an excellent source of protein and Omega-3. Bake it with a mix of vegetables for a simple but healthy meal.

5. **Healthy Snacks**: Keep healthy snacks such as fresh fruit, yogurt, unsalted nuts, or chopped veggies with hummus.

Practical Meal Plans

1. **Meal Prep**: Dedicating a few hours on the weekend to meal prep can help you stick to a healthy eating plan during the week. Cook in large quantities and divide meals into portions that you can store in the refrigerator or freezer.

2. **Balance Your Portions**: Make sure each meal includes a good source of protein, complex carbohydrates (like whole grains or sweet potatoes), and plenty of vegetables.

3. **Variation**: Change foods regularly to ensure a variety of nutrients and maintain interest in eating healthy. Experiment with different vegetables, protein sources, and grains.

4. **Listen to your body**: Eat when you are hungry and stop when you feel full. Avoid eating out of boredom or habit.

5. **Meal Planning**: Take a moment at the beginning of the week to plan your meals. This can help you make more targeted purchases and avoid the dilemma of what to cook every day.

Remember, the secret to healthy eating in old age is not following strict diets but finding joy and satisfaction in eating foods that nourish your body and soul.

3. Yoga for Over 60s

Introduction to Yoga: Benefits for Seniors

Welcome to the chapter dedicated to yoga, an excellent practice that offers immeasurable benefits, especially for those who have reached the age of 60. Yoga is more than just a series of physical exercises; it is a path that unites the body, mind, and spirit, bringing balance and well-being into daily life.

Benefits of Yoga for Seniors

1. **Improved Mobility and Flexibility**: Gentle yoga practices are great for increasing mobility and flexibility, helping to reduce stiffness and pain associated with aging.

2. **Muscle Strengthening**: Through varied postures, yoga helps maintain and build muscle strength, critical to your independence and daily health.

3. **Balance and Stability**: With specific exercises, yoga improves balance, reducing the risk of falls, a common concern in older age.

4. **Stress Management and Mental Wellbeing**: Yoga, breathing, and meditation are powerful tools for managing stress and promoting peace and mental well-being.

Your Yoga Path

In this book, I will guide you through a yoga journey explicitly designed for Seniors, which includes:

- **Basic Yoga Sequences**: You will learn fundamental positions and flows, which are ideal for beginners and adaptable to your needs.

- **30-Day Yoga Program**: A well-structured program with daily exercises designed to gradually introduce you to yoga and help you build a consistent practice.

- **Breathing and Meditation Techniques**: Essential techniques to improve breathing and concentration, critical elements for yoga practice.

- **Post-30 Day Progression**: After the first month, we will explore more advanced exercises and variations to continue developing your practice.

Preparing for Home Practice

To start your yoga practice at home, you will need:

- **A Quiet Space**: Find a quiet place in your home where you can practice without interruptions.

- **A Yoga Mat**: Choose a non-slip mat for comfort and safety.

- **Comfortable Clothing**: Wear clothing that allows for easy mobility.

This chapter is your first step towards a yoga practice that will accompany you to healthy and active aging. Remember, the most important journey is the one we make within ourselves.

Primary Yoga sequences: positions and flows

Welcome to the section dedicated to primary yoga sequences. These locations and flows have been chosen and tailored to be accessible and beneficial to those over 60. These practices will help improve your flexibility, strength, and balance and offer mental and spiritual benefits.

Basic Positions

1. **Mountain Pose (Tadasana) :**

   - Stand your feet together and distribute your weight evenly on both feet.

   - Raise your arms above your head, with palms facing inward.

   - Breathe deeply and hold the position for a few breaths.

2. **Tree Pose (Vrksasana) :**

   - Standing, shift your weight onto one foot.

   - Lift the other foot and rest the sole on the inner calf or above the knee (never on the knee itself).

   - Join your hands in prayer in front of your chest. Hold for a few breaths and then change legs.

3. **Warrior II Pose (Virabhadrasana II) :**

   - With your feet about three feet apart, turn one foot 90 degrees and the other slightly inward.

- Bend your front knee, forming a 90-degree angle, and extend your arms horizontally.

- Look over the fingers of the front hand. Hold for a few breaths, then change sides.

4. **Cat-Cow Pose (Marjaryasana-Bitilasana) :**

- On all fours, with your knees under your hips and your hands under your shoulders.

- Inhaling, lower your abdomen towards the floor, raising your head and tail (Cow).

- Exhaling, round your back towards the ceiling, lowering your head (Cat).

- Continue moving between these two positions for several breaths.

5. **Child's Pose (Balasana) :**

- Sit on your heels, bend forward, bringing your forehead to the ground.

- Extend your arms in front of you or at your sides.

- Relax in this position for deep breaths.

6. **Downward Facing Dog Position (Adho Mukha Svanasana) :**

- Start on all fours with your hands slightly before your shoulders.

- Lift your hips up and back, extending your arms and legs.

- Try to lower your heels toward the floor for a good stretch.

- Hold your head in your arms and hold the position briefly.

7. **Warrior Pose I (Virabhadrasana I)** :

- From a standing position, take a big step back with one foot.

- Bend your front knee to 90 degrees, keeping your back foot flat and rotated slightly outward.

- Raise your arms above your head, keeping your shoulders relaxed.

- Hold the position for a few breaths, then change sides.

Basic Flows

A yoga flow connects different poses through movement and breathing. Here's a simple flow to try:

1. **Simple Sun Salutation Flow** :

   - Start in Mountain Pose.

   - Inhaling, raise your arms above your head.

   - Exhale, bend forward from the waist and your hands toward the floor (bend your knees slightly if necessary).

   - Inhaling, raise your torso halfway, back straight.

   - Exhale, return to a standing position and return your hands to the prayer position.

2. **Warrior Flow** :

   - Start in Mountain Pose.

   - With a wide stride, move into Warrior II Pose.

   - After a few breaths, bring your hands to the ground and return to your feet.

   - Repeat on the other side.

3. **Warrior Stance Flow** :

   - Start in Mountain Pose.

- With a wide stride, move into Warrior I Stance.

- Raise your arms above your head and hold for a few breaths.

- Move into Warrior II Pose, rotating your torso to the side and extending your arms.

- Hold a few breaths, then return to Mountain Pose and repeat on the other side.

4. **Relaxation and Stretching Flow** :

- Start sitting with your legs crossed.

- Inhaling, raise your arms above your head.

- Exhaling, bend forward from the waist, trying to touch the floor before you.

- Hold for a few breaths, then slowly return to sitting.

- Repeat the flow for a few cycles.

Remember to move slowly and listen to your body. If a position causes pain, try a variation or move on to the next. These sequences are the starting point for building your yoga practice.

30 day Yoga program with daily exercises

Week 1: Fundamentals and Breathing

- **Day 1** :

  - Start with 5 minutes of deep breathing in Mountain Pose (Tadasana).

  - Proceed with 10 minutes of Cat-Cow (Marjaryasana-Bitilasana) to warm up the spine.

- **Day 2** :

  - Practice Tree Pose (Vrksasana) on each side for 5 minutes to improve balance.

  - Conclude with 5 minutes of Child's Pose (Balasana) for relaxation.

- **Day 3** :

  - Introduce Warrior II Pose (Virabhadrasana II) and hold for 30 seconds on each side.

  - Relax with Child's Pose for 5 minutes.

- **Day 4** :

  - Repeat the sequence from Day 2.

- **Day 5** :

- Combine the learned positions in a fluid sequence, switching between them every 2 minutes.

- **Day 6** :

  - Repeat the Day 3 sequence.

- **Day 7** :

  - Day of rest or guided meditation.

Week 2: Building Strength and Flexibility

- **Day 8-14** :

  - Each day, begin with 5 minutes of Mountain Pose, focusing on your breathing.

  - Gradually introduce Downward Facing Dog (Adho Mukha Svanasana), holding the position for 1 minute.

  - Alternate between Warrior I and II, holding each position for 1 minute on each side.

  - Each session should end with 5 minutes of Child's Pose to relax.

Week 3: Dynamic Flows and Balance

- **Day 15-21** :

- Begin with a modified Sun Salutation sequence, performing it for 10 minutes.

- Integrate Warrior I and II into a smooth flow, moving from one position to another for 10 minutes.

- Finish with 5 minutes of meditation or mindful breathing.

Week 4: Integration and Complete Practice

- **Day 22-28** :

  - Practice a complete sequence that integrates all the positions learned, starting with the Sun Salutation and including Warrior I and II, Downward Facing Dog, and Tree.

  - Dedicate at least 20 minutes to this practice.

- **Day 29** :

  - The yoga session is dedicated to stretching and relaxation, mainly using the Child and Cat-Cow Pose.

- **Day 30** :

- A celebratory practice, retracing all the positions learned and dedicating time to reflect on the progress.

Tips for Practice

- Practice in a quiet and comfortable place.

- Listen to your body: if a position is too difficult, adapt it or move on to the next.

- Maintain regular, deep breathing during practice.

- Use accessories such as pillows or yoga blocks as needed for comfort.

This program will guide you through a progressive yoga practice suited to your needs and abilities. Remember, the yoga journey is personal and flexible; Always adapt the training to your needs.

Breathing and meditation techniques

Incorporating breathing and meditation techniques into your yoga practice is essential to achieving complete well-being. These techniques enhance physical practice and profoundly benefit the mind and spirit, especially in older age. Here are some fundamental methods you can explore:

Breathing Techniques (Pranayama)

1. **Diaphragmatic Breathing (Abdominal Breathing)** :

   - Sit comfortably or lie on your back.

   - Place one hand on your abdomen and the other on your chest.

   - Breathe slowly through your nose, focusing on expanding your abdomen rather than lifting your chest.

   - Exhale slowly, feeling your abdomen lower.

   - Continue for 5-10 minutes, focusing on the movement of your abdomen.

2. **Three-Part Breathing (Dirga Pranayama)** :

   - In a sitting or lying position, begin to breathe deeply.

   - Imagine filling the lower abdomen first, then the central part of the chest, and finally the upper part near the collarbones.

   - Exhale in the same order: first, empty the air from the upper part of the chest, then from the center, and finally from the lower abdomen.

- Repeat for several breaths, trying to make each
  part equally long.

Meditation techniques

1. **Awareness Meditation (Mindfulness)** :

   - Find a quiet place and sit with your back straight.

   - Close your eyes and focus on breathing, noticing
     each inhalation and exhalation.

   - When your mind wanders, gently bring your
     attention to your breathing.

   - Continue for 5-15 minutes.

2. **Guided Meditation** :

   - Use guided meditation recordings or participate in
     age-specific guided meditation classes.

   - Follow the spoken instructions, allowing your
     mind to relax and be guided through images and
     sensations.

3. **Walking Meditation** :

   - Find a quiet path where you can walk without
     distractions.

- Concentrate on the movement of your feet and the rhythm of your step, synchronizing it with your breathing.

- Whenever your mind wanders, gently bring it back to the movement of your feet and breathing.

Integrating Breathing and Meditation into Yoga Practice

- Before starting your yoga session, do diaphragmatic breathing to center yourself and prepare yourself.

- While practicing the asanas (positions), maintain constant and deep breathing, using three-part breathing.

- Conclude each yoga session with a 5-10 minute meditation, choosing the technique that best suits you at that moment.

Remember, regular practice is the key. Even just a few minutes a day of breathing and meditation can significantly benefit your physical and mental health.

Post-30 Day Progression: Advanced Exercises and Variations

After completing the 30-day yoga program, you may wonder how to continue and deepen your practice. Here are some ideas for post-30-day progressions, including advanced variations and new exercises to incorporate into your daily routine.

Advanced Exercises and Variations

1. **Triangle Pose (Trikonasana) :**

   - From a standing position, spread your feet about one meter apart.

   - Extend your arms horizontally, turning one foot 90 degrees and the other slightly inward.

   - Bend laterally towards the foot that points outwards, trying to touch the ankle, calf, or knee.

   - Look up at the hand above your head.

   - Hold for a few breaths, then change sides.

2. **Fisherman's Pose (Matsyasana) :**

   - Sit with your legs crossed.

   - Rest on your hands, bend your elbows, and slowly lower yourself to the ground, arching your back.

   - Let your head hang back, opening your chest.

   - Hold for a few breaths.

3. **Chair Pose (Utkatasana) :**

- Standing in Mountain Pose, bend your knees as if you were sitting in an imaginary chair.

- Raise your arms above your head, keeping your shoulders relaxed.

- Hold the position for a few breaths.

4. **Variations on Sun Salutation** :

- Include new poses like Downward Facing Dog and Warrior I in your Sun Salutation sequences, increasing the complexity of the flow.

5. **One-Leg Balance (Vrksasana Variations)** :

- In Tree Pose, lift the foot higher on the opposite thigh.

- For an added challenge, try closing your eyes for a few seconds.

Tips for Progression

- **Listen to your body**: Never force yourself into a position that causes pain or is too difficult.

- **Regular Practice**: Continue to practice regularly, gradually increasing the length or complexity of your sessions.

- **Explore New Classes**: Consider taking advanced yoga classes or workshops to explore new techniques and styles.

- **Integrate Meditation and Breathing**: Continue to practice deep breathing and meditation as part of your yoga routine.

Deepening of Spiritual Practice

- **Yoga Nidra**: Explore deep relaxation practices like Yoga Nidra for greater inner awareness.

- **Study Yoga Philosophy**: Read yoga texts or participate in study groups to deepen your understanding of yoga philosophy.

Remember, progression in yoga is not just physical. It also includes spiritual and mental growth. Celebrate your progress and enjoy the ongoing journey of exploration and discovery.

4. Stretching and Flexibility for Over 60s

Benefits of Stretching for Seniors

Stretching offers numerous benefits for seniors, significantly contributing to improving the quality of life at this stage. Here are some key benefits of stretching for seniors :

1. **Improved Flexibility and Joint Mobility**: As we age, joints become stiffer and less flexible. Stretching helps maintain flexibility, reduce the risk of injury, and improve joint mobility, making daily activities such as bending, turning, and reaching objects easier.

2. **Increased Blood Circulation**: Regular stretching improves blood circulation, which is essential for overall health. Good circulation helps deliver oxygen and vital nutrients to various tissues in the body, promoting healing and reducing the risk of muscle cramps.

3. **Reduced Pain and Muscle Tension**: Seniors often suffer from muscle pain and stiffness due to inactivity or chronic diseases such as arthritis. Stretching can help relieve these uncomfortable feelings by improving flexibility and reducing muscle tension.

4. **Improved Posture**: Your posture can worsen as you age, leading to pain and balance problems. Stretching helps strengthen postural muscles, helps maintain an upright posture, and prevents back pain.

5. **Fall Prevention**: Stretching improves balance and coordination, two critical factors in preventing falls, a standard risk for seniors. Keeping your muscles flexible and responsive is essential to maintaining balance.

6. **Improved Mental Health**: Stretching can also positively affect mental health. It is a relaxing activity that can reduce stress and anxiety, improve mood, and promote quality sleep.

7. **Increase in Personal Autonomy**: By maintaining good flexibility and mobility, Seniors can preserve their autonomy and ability to carry out daily activities without excessive dependence on others.

8. **Ease and Accessibility**: Stretching is a physical activity that can be done almost anywhere and requires no special equipment. It is easily adaptable to individual abilities, making it ideal for people of all ages and physical conditions.

To maximize the benefits of stretching, it is essential to perform the exercises correctly, hold each stretch for at least 15-30 seconds, and practice a routine. It is also advisable to consult a qualified physiotherapist or fitness instructor to develop a tailored stretching program, mainly if health concerns or physical limitations exist.

Basic and advanced stretching exercises

Stretching exercises are essential for maintaining flexibility, improving mobility, and reducing the risk of injury, especially in Seniors. This guide offers a series of basic and advanced stretching exercises designed to be performed comfortably at home. Whether you are a beginner or already have experience with stretching, these exercises can be adapted to your needs and abilities.

General consideration

1. **Heating**: Preparing your body with a proper warm-up is essential before starting any stretching session. Here are some warm-up exercises suitable for seniors :

- **Walk in Place or Light March**: Walk in place or do a light march for 3-5 minutes to work your entire body and increase your heart rate.

- **Arm Rotations**: Standing with your arms extended to your sides, perform circular arm movements for 1-2 minutes to warm up your shoulders and upper body.

- **Head and Neck Rotation**: Perform slow, controlled neck rotations, moving the head up and down, left and right, and in circular motions to release tension.

- **Leg Raises**: Sitting in a chair or standing, lift one leg at a time, bending the knee toward your chest to warm up the leg and hip muscles.

- **Pelvic Rotations**: With your hands on your hips, make circular motions with your pelvis to warm up your abdominal and lower back muscles.

- **Light Dynamic Stretching**: To increase joint mobility, perform light, dynamic stretching movements, such as arm swings or sideways body tilts.

These warm-up exercises should be performed with slow, controlled movements, avoiding jerking or forcing. The total duration of the warm-up can vary between 5 and 10 minutes, depending on your comfort level and physical ability. The goal is to leave yourself energized and ready to stretch, not tired.

2. **Breathing**: Maintain deep, controlled breathing during exercises.

3. **Listen to Your Body**: Avoid movements that cause pain or discomfort.

4. **Regularity**: Practice the exercises regularly to obtain maximum benefit.

5. **Gradual Progression**: Increase the intensity and duration of exercises over time.

Basic Stretching Exercises

1. **Neck Stretch** :

   - Sitting or standing, slowly lower your head towards your chest and tilt it back.

   - Turn your head left and right, holding each position for 15-20 seconds.

2. **Shoulder Stretch** :

   - Bring one arm horizontally across your body, using the other arm to pull gently.

   - Hold for 20-30 seconds on each side.

3. **Upper Arm and Back Stretch** :

   - Bring your arms behind your back, interlace your fingers, and lift your arms to stretch your upper back.

   - Maintain for 20-30 seconds.

4. **Calf Stretch** :

- Face a wall. With one leg behind and the other in front, push against the wall while keeping your back heel on the ground.

- Hold each leg for 20-30 seconds.

5. **Quadriceps Stretch** :

- Standing, bend one knee and bring your heel towards your buttocks, grasping your ankle with your hand.

- Hold each leg for 20-30 seconds.

Advanced Stretching Exercises

1. **Advanced Leg Stretching (Toe Touch)** :

- Sitting on the ground with your legs extended, leaning forward to touch your toes.

- Hold for 45-60 seconds.

2. **Torso Twists** :

- Sitting on the floor with one leg bent and the other extended, rotate your torso towards the bent leg.

- Hold for 45-60 seconds each side.

3. **Advanced Hip Stretch (Pigeon Pose)** :

- From an all-fours position, bring one knee forward and the other leg extended back.

- Lean your torso forward for a deeper stretch.

- Hold for 45-60 seconds each side.

4. **Pelvic Bridge** :

- Lying on your back, with your knees bent and feet on the ground, lift your hips into a bridge.

- Hold for 30-45 seconds.

These stretching exercises are designed to be inclusive and accessible to people of all ages and ability levels. Regularly performing these exercises can significantly improve flexibility, mobility, and overall quality of life. Remember to proceed cautiously, listen to your body, and enjoy the benefits of a more active and healthy lifestyle.

Daily stretching routines

Establishing a daily stretching routine is vital to maintaining flexibility, reducing the risk of injury, and improving overall well-being, especially in Seniors. Here is a stretching routine that can be easily integrated into daily life.

Morning: Muscle awakening

- **Neck Stretch**: Stand or sit, lower your head toward your chest, and tilt it back, left and right. Hold each position for 15-20 seconds.

- **Arm Rotations**: Raise your arms to the side and rotate them in circular motions for 1-2 minutes.

- **Leg Stretch**: Sitting on the edge of the bed, extend one leg and lean forward, trying to touch your feet. Hold each leg for 20-30 seconds.

Afternoon: Activation and Maintenance

- **Shoulder Stretch**: Bring one arm horizontally across your body, using the other arm to pull it gently. Hold for 20-30 seconds on each side.

- **Calf Stretch**: Lean against a wall with one leg in front and the other behind. Bend your front leg and push your back heel towards the floor. Hold each leg for 20-30 seconds.

Evening: Relaxation and relaxation

- **Torso Twists**: Sitting on the floor with one leg extended and the other bent, rotate your torso toward your bent leg. Hold each side for 45-60 seconds.

- **Pelvic Bridge**: Lying on your back, with your knees bent and feet on the ground, lift your hips into a bridge. Hold for 30-45 seconds.

- **Upper Arm and Back Stretch**: Interlace your fingers behind your back and lift your arms, lengthening your upper back. Maintain for 20-30 seconds.

General consideration

- **Duration**: Dedicate approximately 10-15 minutes for each stretching session.

- **Consistency**: Practice your stretching routine every day to maximize benefits.

- **Listen to the Body**: Don't force the movements and stop if you feel pain.

- **Breathing**: Maintain deep, regular breathing during exercises.

This daily stretching routine can be adapted to suit individual needs and abilities. Regularity and consistency in stretching are more important than the intensity of the exercises. Over time, these exercises can help improve mobility, reduce pain, and increase overall well-being.

30-day stretching program

The following 30-day stretching program is designed to gradually help improve flexibility, reduce muscle tension, and improve overall well-being. The routine intensifies each week, allowing the body to adapt and improve.

Week 1: Introduction to Stretching

- **Frequency**: Stretching every day.

- **Duration**: 10 minutes per session.

- **Focus**: Basic exercises such as stretching the neck, shoulders, calves, and quadriceps.

- **Goal**: Get used to a daily stretching routine.

Week 2: Base Construction

- **Frequency**: Every day.

- **Duration**: Increase to 15 minutes per session.

- **Additions**: Introduce light dynamic stretching and increase the hold time for each stretch to 30 seconds.

- **Objective**: Improve essential flexibility and stretching tolerance.

Week 3: Increased Intensity

- **Frequency**: Every day.

- **Duration**: Keep at 15 minutes.

- **Additions**: Include trunk rotations and pelvic bridge. Begin introducing more advanced stretches, such as toe touch and pigeon pose.

- **Goal**: Begin exploring a more excellent range of motion.

Week 4: Deepening and Consolidation

- **Frequency**: Every day.

- **Duration**: Extend to 20 minutes per session.

- **Focus**: Continue with all previous exercises, emphasizing advanced stretches.

- **Objective**: Consolidate your stretching routine and further improve flexibility.

General consideration

- **Listen to the Body**: If an exercise causes pain, it is vital to stop and consult a professional.

- **Consistency**: Maintaining your daily routine to see progress is essential.

- **Breathing**: Make sure you breathe deeply and regularly during the exercises.

- **Warm-up**: Start each session with a short warm-up to prepare your muscles.

Upon completing the 30-day program, you should notice an improvement in overall flexibility, a reduction in muscle tension, and an increase in well-being. This program can be adapted or repeated to improve or maintain the benefits obtained.

Post-30 Day Progression: Advanced Techniques

After completing the 30-day stretching program, you must challenge your body and progress to more advanced stretching techniques. This progression phase helps maintain and further improve flexibility, strength, and overall well-being.

Increase in Duration and Intensity

- **Duration**: Extend each stretching session to 25-30 minutes.

- **Intensity**: Gradually increase the intensity of the stretches, holding the positions for more extended periods, up to 60 seconds.

Advanced Stretching Techniques

- **Deep Leg Stretch**: Sitting with your legs extended, bend forward from the pelvis, trying to lower your chest towards your legs as much as possible.

- **Balasana (Child's Pose)**: From an all-fours position, sit on your heels with your arms extended forward and your head on the ground. This position stretches your back and hips.

- **Anjaneyasana (Low Lunge)**: Standing, take a big step back with one leg, place your back knee on the ground, and tilt your pelvis forward to lengthen your hip.

- **Camel Pose (Ustrasana)**: On your knees, bend backward to reach your heels with your hands, lengthening your chest and abdomen.

- **Advanced Pigeon Pose**: Starting from basic Pigeon Pose, lean forward to lengthen your hips and lower back further.

Integration of Yoga and Pilates

- Integrate elements of yoga and Pilates to increase flexibility, strength, and body control.

- Exercises such as Plank, Cat-Cow, and Warrior Poses can be added to improve core strength and stability.

Recovery and Self-Healing

- **Cool-down**: Conclude each session with a 5-10 minute cool-down, deep breathing and muscle relaxation.

- **Self-care**: Use techniques like guided relaxation or meditation to help your body and mind relax after exercise.

Progress Monitoring

- Track your weekly progress to see improvements in flexibility and ease of performing exercises.

Consultation of Experts

- Consider consulting a physical therapist or qualified yoga instructor to ensure advanced exercises are performed safely and effectively.

This post-30-day progression phase is ideal for those looking to deepen their stretching practice and improve their physical health. To avoid injury, listening to your body and proceeding cautiously is essential, especially with advanced techniques. These advanced exercises can significantly benefit your physical and mental health with regular practice.

5. Pilates for Over 60s

Introduction to Pilates: health benefits

Pilates is an exercise system that emphasizes improving flexibility, strength, and body awareness without necessarily building muscle mass. This practice, developed by Joseph Pilates in the early 20th century, has become famous worldwide for its many health benefits. Below are some of the main benefits that Pilates offers:

1. Improved Flexibility

- Pilates constantly lengthens the muscles and increases the length of the muscles and the range of motion of the joints.

2. Core Strengthening

- One of the main goals of Pilates is strengthening the core muscles (abdomen, back, and hips), which is essential for good posture and balance.

3. Improved Posture

- Thanks to working on the core and awareness of one's body, Pilates helps improve posture, reducing the risk of pain and problems related to incorrect posture.

4. Prevention and Reduction of Back Pain

- Strengthening and stretching your core muscles, especially those around your lower back, can prevent or reduce back pain.

5. Increased Muscle Strength

- Pilates involves resistance and strength exercises, helping to build strong, balanced muscles.

6. Improved Balance and Coordination

- Pilates requires precise body control and fluid movement, thus improving balance and coordination.

7. Stress Reduction and Improved Concentration

- The practice requires concentration and controlled breathing, contributing to the reduction of stress and increased concentration.

8. Adaptability to Individuals

- Pilates exercises can be modified to meet individual needs, making it accessible to everyone, regardless of age or fitness level.

9. Increase in Energy

- Pilates stimulates circulation and increases flexibility and strength, contributing to more incredible energy and vitality.

10. Improved Body Awareness

- The practice of Pilates helps to develop a greater awareness of one's body, its movements, and its abilities.

Introducing Pilates can offer a transformative path to overall health and well-being. With its emphasis on a balanced workout that engages the mind, body, and spirit, Pilates is an effective method for improving physical fitness and increasing psychological and emotional well-being.

Pilates exercises for strength and posture

Pilates is an effective method for building strength and improving posture, particularly in the core. Here are some Pilates exercises focused on these aspects:

1. The Hundred

- **Initial position**: Lie on your back, knees bent at 90 degrees, head and shoulders raised off the ground.

- **Execution**: Extend your arms at your sides, palms facing down. Pump your arms up and down in small motions, breathing deeply for 100 counts.

- **Benefits**: Strengthens the core and improves breathing capacity.

2. The Roll-Up

- **Initial position**: Lie on your back, arms stretched above your head, and legs extended.

- **Execution**: Inhale, raise your arms towards the ceiling, then exhale, slowly roll your spine into a sitting position, reaching towards your toes. Return to the starting position with control.

- **Benefits**: Improves spinal flexibility and strengthens the abdominals.

3. The Swan

- **Initial position**: Lying on your stomach, arms bent with hands near your shoulders.

- **Execution**: Slowly lift your chest off the ground by extending your arms, maintaining a slight curve in your lower back. Return to the starting position with control.

- **Benefits**: Strengthens the back and improves posture.

4. Single Leg Circles (One Leg Circles)

- **Initial position**: Lie on your back, one leg extending towards the ceiling and the other on the ground.

- **Execution**: Move the elevated leg in small controlled circles, keeping the pelvis stable. Repeat in both directions, then change legs.

- **Benefits**: Improves core stability and hip mobility.

5. Spine Stretch Forward

- **Initial position**: Sitting with legs extended, feet slightly wider than shoulders.

- **Execution**: Inhale, lengthen the spine upwards, exhale, bend forward from the pelvis, and try to reach the feet with the hands.

- **Benefits**: Stretches the spine and improves posture.

6. Pelvic Curl (Pelvic Curl)

- **Initial position**: Lie on your back, feet on the ground and shoulder-width apart, arms at the sides.

- **Execution**: Slowly lift your pelvis off the floor, forming a straight line from shoulders to knees. Return to the starting position by rolling the spine vertebra by vertebra.

- **Benefits**: Strengthens the core, glutes, and back, improving pelvic stability.

General consideration

- Perform each exercise with controlled, fluid movements.

- Keep breathing coordinated with movement.

- Listen to your body; don't force movements if they cause pain.

- Start with a few repetitions, gradually increasing.

These Pilates exercises help build strength, especially in the core, and improve posture and body alignment. Regular practice can lead to a significant improvement in overall physical health and well-being.

30-day Pilates program

This 30-day program is designed to gradually introduce Pilates exercises, build core strength, and improve posture. Each week, the program intensifies slightly, allowing the body to adapt and progressively improve.

Week 1: Introduction and Fundamentals

- **Frequency**: Practice Pilates for 20 minutes daily, five days a week.

- **Focus**: Concentrate on basic exercises such as The Hundred, Pelvic Curl, and The Roll-Up.

- **Objective**: Familiarize yourself with the fundamental principles of Pilates, such as core control and breathing.

Week 2: Building Core Strength

- **Frequency**: Increase to 25 minutes per day.

- **Additions**: Introduce exercises such as single-leg circles and spine stretch forward.

- **Goal**: Start building core strength and improve flexibility.

Week 3: Integration and Fluency

- **Frequency**: Maintain 25 minutes per day.

- **Additions**: Add exercises like The Swan and other stretching and strengthening exercises.

- **Objective**: Integrate new movements, improving fluidity and control.

Week 4: Intensification and Depth

- **Frequency**: Increase to 30 minutes per day.

- **Focus**: Combining all the exercises learned, increasing the number of repetitions and complexity.

- **Objective**: Challenge with more complex exercises, strengthening the entire body and improving posture.

General consideration

- **Warm-up**: Begin each session with a short warm-up to prepare your body.

- **Consistency**: It is essential to maintain regular practice to see progress.

- **Listening to the Body**: Modify the exercises according to your needs, and don't hesitate to take breaks when necessary.

- **Cool-down**: Conclude each session with relaxation and stretching exercises.

At the end of the 30-day program, you should notice an improvement in your core strength, flexibility, posture, and body awareness. This program can be adapted or repeated to maintain or further improve the benefits obtained.

Tips for avoiding injuries

Avoiding injuries during exercise, whether Pilates, stretching, or any other activity, is crucial to maintaining a healthy and active lifestyle, especially as you age. Here are some critical tips for preventing injuries:

1. Adequate warm-up

- Proper warm-ups are essential before starting any physical activity. This may include walking in place, joint rotations, or dynamic stretching to prepare the body for exercise.

2. Listen to your body

- Pay attention to your body's signals. Stopping and evaluating the situation is essential if you feel pain or discomfort. Don't ignore pain, which is a warning signal from the body.

3. Gradually Increase the Intensity

- Gradually increase the intensity and duration of the exercises to avoid overloading the muscles and joints. This is especially important for those new to physical activity or returning after a break.

4. Use Correct Technique

- Make sure you perform each exercise with the correct technique. Consider working with a qualified instructor, especially when starting a new type of workout or performing complex movements.

5. Wear Appropriate Equipment

- Use appropriate equipment, such as shoes for your activity, to support your body and reduce the risk of injury.

6. Hydration and Nutrition

- Keep your body well-hydrated and nourished. Water and essential nutrients are crucial for optimal muscle function and injury prevention.

7. Avoid Overexertion

- Give your body time to rest and recover between workouts. Overexertion can lead to injuries and fatigue.

8. Cool-down and Post-Workout Stretching

- Conclude each training session with a proper cool-down and stretching. This helps reduce muscle stiffness and promotes repair and recovery.

9. Pay Attention to the Environment

- Make sure the training area is safe, free of obstacles, and has a stable surface to avoid falls and slips.

10. Listen to Health Professionals

- If you have any pre-existing conditions or health concerns, consult a doctor or physical therapist before starting a new exercise program.

By following these tips, you can significantly reduce your risk of injury and enjoy safe and beneficial physical activity. Remember that prevention is the key to a long and healthy career in exercise.

Post-30-day progression: more intense exercises and variations

After completing an initial 30-day Pilates program, continuing to challenge the body with more intense exercises and variations is essential. This helps you maintain interest and engagement and improves your strength, flexibility, and overall health.

Intensified Exercises

- **Control Balance**: From a prone position, lift your legs towards the ceiling and above your head, maintaining control and balance.

- **Jackknife**: This is similar to Control Balance but with a more dynamic movement of the legs up and over the head.

- **Teaser Variations**: To increase the intensity, perform the Teaser with variations, such as extended legs or a rotating motion.

Variations of Existing Exercises

- **The Hundred with Low Legs**: Perform The Hundred with your legs lower to the floor to increase the intensity of the core work.

- **Plank Variations: Introduce variations in the** plank position, such as the side plank or one-leg raised plank, to increase the challenge.

- **Roll-Up with Ball**: Use a Pilates ball during the Roll-Up to improve control and stability.

Adding Equipment

- **Magic Circle**: Use the Magic Circle to add resistance in exercises like Side Leg Lifts or Arm Presses.

- **Pilates Ball**: To increase the difficulty and improve balance, integrate a small ball into exercises such as the Bridge or Prone Leg Lift.

- **Resistance Bands**: Use resistance bands in exercises like Arm Stretches or Leg Extensions for more intense work.

Focus on Fluidity and Control

- Increase fluidity and control in movements, making each exercise more continuous and connected to the next.

- Keep your focus on the quality of movement rather than quantity.

Increased Complexity

- Combine exercises to create longer, more complex sequences.

- Experiment with more difficult transitions between exercises.

Progression in Pilates is not limited to increasing physical difficulty but also includes deepening body awareness and improving control and precision. Exploring new challenges and variations will help keep the practice fresh, exciting, and beneficial to physical and mental health.

6. Cardio Fitness for Over 60s

Cardio training: benefits for seniors

Cardio or cardiovascular training is essential for seniors, offering numerous physical and mental health benefits. Here are some of the main advantages:

1. Improved Heart Health

- Cardiovascular training helps strengthen the heart, improving its ability to pump blood more efficiently and reducing the risk of heart disease.

2. Increased Lung Capacity

- Regular cardio activities increase lung capacity, improving the body's oxygenation and respiratory efficiency.

3. Weight Control

- Cardio training helps you burn calories and maintain a healthy body weight, reducing the risk of obesity, type 2 diabetes, and other related conditions.

4. Reduction of Blood Pressure

- Regular exercise can help reduce high blood pressure, a significant risk factor for stroke and heart disease.

5. Improved Muscle Strength

- While cardio training primarily focuses on heart and lung health, it also helps maintain and improve muscle strength, especially in the legs.

6. Increase Energy and Reduce Fatigue

- Regular cardiovascular exercise improves stamina and energy levels, helping seniors feel less tired daily.

7. Improved Metabolism

- Cardio training can increase your metabolic rate, making it easier to manage weight and improving the body's energy efficiency.

8. Prevention and Management of Depression

- Regular exercise has been linked to reduced symptoms of depression and anxiety, thanks to the production of endorphins, chemicals that improve mood.

9. Improved Mobility and Reduced Risk of Falls

- Cardio training improves balance, coordination, and mobility, reducing the risk of falls and improving the ability to carry out daily activities.

10. Improved Sleep

- Seniors who regularly exercise cardio often report improved sleep quality, including ease of falling asleep and deeper sleep.

Incorporate cardio training into your exercise routine. Seniors can significantly improve overall health, well-being, and quality of life. However, Seniors need to consult a doctor before starting any new exercise program, especially if they have pre-existing conditions or have been inactive for a prolonged period.

Low-impact cardio exercises

These low-impact cardio exercises are ideal for seniors over 60, providing a safe and effective way to maintain cardiovascular health without leaving home. Here is a detailed description to make each exercise easily understandable:

1. March on the spot

- **How to do it**: Stand with free space around you. Raise your knees one at a time, simulating a march.

- **Key Points**: Keep your back straight. Raise your knees as high as you can comfortably.

- **Recommended duration**: Start with 5 minutes, gradually increasing.

2. Step-Up on Step

- **How to**: Use a low step or the first step of a staircase. Place one foot on the step and lift yourself, then step down and repeat with the other foot.

- **Key Points**: Maintain balance and use your leg to lift your body; don't push too hard with your leg on the ground.

- **Recommended duration**: 5-10 minutes, depending on capacity.

3. Chair exercises

- **How to do it**: Sit on a stable chair without armrests. Perform mini-squats while sitting and lifting slightly, or lift one leg at a time, keeping it straight.

- **Key Points**: Keep your back straight. Use your leg muscles for movements.

- **Recommended repetitions**: 10-15 per leg or per squat.

4. Low Impact Dance

- **How to do it**: Put on some music and move freely in the available space with light and controlled movements.

- **Key Points**: Avoid jumping or sudden movements. Focus on smooth movements that increase your heart rate.

- **Recommended duration**: 10-15 minutes.

5. Arm Exercises with Water Bottles

- **How To**: Hold a bottle of water in each hand. Perform front and lateral arm raises.

- **Key Points**: Keep your arms straight but not locked. Raise to shoulder height.

- **Recommended repetitions**: 10-15 for each movement.

6. Lateral Walk

- **How to do it**: Stand with your legs slightly apart. Move sideways to one side of the room and then to the other.

- **Key Points**: Take small steps, maintaining balance. Add the use of your arms for greater cardio involvement.

- **Recommended duration**: 5-10 minutes.

7. Dynamic Stretching Exercises

- **How to Do It**: Combine stretching movements with cardio elements, such as raising your arms or leaning your body to the side while walking in place.

- **Key Points**: Focus on smooth, controlled movements. Synchronize breathing with movement.

- **Recommended duration**: 5-10 minutes.

Performance Tips

- Start each exercise slowly, gradually increasing the intensity.

- Take breaks when necessary and drink water to maintain hydration.

- Listen to your body: stop if you feel pain or excessive fatigue.

These exercises are ideal for Seniors over 60, as they offer an effective cardio workout with reduced impact on the joints and can be performed comfortably and safely at home.

30-day cardio program

This 30-day program is designed to help Seniors over 60 gradually increase their cardiovascular capacity and improve their overall health. The program is based on gradually increasing intensity and duration, ensuring a safe and progressive workout.

Week 1: Introduction and Adaptation

- **Goal**: Familiarize yourself with low-impact cardio exercises.

- **Routine**: Alternate walking in place, low-impact dancing, and lateral walking.

- **Duration**: Start with 10 minutes a day, five days a week.

Week 2: Increased Intensity

- **Objective**: Gradually increase the intensity of the exercises.

- **Routine**: Introduce arm exercises with water bottles and step-ups on steps.

- **Duration**: Increase to 15 minutes daily, maintaining five days a week.

Week 3: Variation and Resistance

- **Objective**: Introduce variations in exercises to keep training stimulating.

- **Routine**: Add variations in movements while dancing and marching in place. Include dynamic stretching.

- **Duration**: Bring to 20 minutes a day.

Week 4: Consolidation and Intensification

- **Goal**: Strengthen your cardio routine with a greater emphasis on resistance.

- **Routine**: Combine all the exercises learned with smooth transitions from one to the next.

- **Duration**: Increase to 25-30 minutes per day.

General Tips

- **Listen to the Body**: Pay attention to how you feel during exercise and take breaks if necessary.

- **Hydration**: Be sure to drink water before, during and after exercise.

- **Warm-up and Cool-down**: Begin each session with a light warm-up and conclude with a light cool-down and stretching.

- **Progression**: Increase the intensity and duration of the exercises gradually.

This 30-day program is designed to be flexible and adaptable to the individual capabilities of Seniors over 60. Upon completing the program, you should notice an improvement in cardiovascular endurance, energy, and general well-being. Furthermore, these exercises can be a solid foundation for maintaining regular physical activity after completing the program.

Strategies to improve cardiovascular health

Improving cardiovascular health is essential for seniors over 60. Here are some effective strategies that go beyond exercise:

1. Healthy and Balanced Diet

- **Focus**: Consume a diet rich in fruits, vegetables, whole grains, lean proteins and healthy fats.

- **Tips**: Limit salt, added sugars, and saturated fats consumption.

2. Maintain a Healthy Body Weight

- **Strategy**: Balance calorie intake with physical activity.

- **Tips**: Monitor your weight regularly and consult a nutritionist for personalized advice.

3. Stress Management

- **Techniques**: Practice relaxation techniques such as meditation, yoga, or tai chi.

- **Benefits**: Reducing stress can lower blood pressure and improve cardiovascular health.

4. Stop Smoking

- **Importance**: Smoking is a significant risk factor for cardiovascular disease.

- **Support**: Seek help programs to quit smoking, which may include counseling or medical treatment.

5. Regular monitoring of blood pressure and cholesterol

- **Monitoring**: Measure blood pressure regularly and have periodic cholesterol checks.

- **Action**: Consult a doctor for targeted interventions in high values.

6. Reduction of Alcohol Consumption

- **Guidance**: Limit alcohol consumption to moderate levels.

- **Effect**: Excessive alcohol consumption can increase blood pressure and the risk of heart disease.

7. Sleep well

- **Importance**: Quality sleep is essential for heart health.

- **Tips**: Create a relaxing evening routine and maintain a comfortable sleep environment.

8. Maintain Regular Physical Activity

- **Exercise**: Incorporate low-impact cardio, strength, and flexibility into your weekly routine.

- **Benefits**: Helps keep the heart strong and improve circulation.

9. Socialization and Recreational Activities

- **Benefits**: Maintaining social connections and participating in group activities helps reduce stress and improve mental well-being.

- **Options**: Join clubs and walking groups or participate in community events.

Adopting a healthy lifestyle is crucial for cardiovascular health, especially for seniors over 60. A balanced diet, regular exercise, stress management, and health monitoring can significantly improve heart health and quality of life.

Post-30-day progression: introduction of new activities

After an initial 30-day program focused on low-impact cardio exercises, Seniors over 60 can introduce new cardio activities to keep the routine stimulating and continue to improve their cardiovascular health. Here is a detailed description of these activities:

1. March with knee raise and arm movement

- **How to Do It**: March in place, raising your knees as high as possible. Then, move your arms dynamically, raising them above your head or moving them back and forth.

- **Duration**: 10-15 minutes, gradually increasing the pace.

2. Low-Intensity Aerobic Dance

- **How to**: Watch a low-impact aerobic dance video focusing on fluid, continuous movements that raise your heart rate.

- **Tip**: Choose simple dance styles like line dancing or adapted folk dances.

- **Duration**: Start with 10 minutes, gradually increasing.

3. Step Exercises Using a Low-Step

- **How To**: Use a low-step or stable platform. Go up and down the step with alternating legs.

- **Points of Attention**: Keep your back straight and focus on stability.

- **Duration**: Do 2-3 sets of 5 minutes each.

4. Arm exercises with water bottles or light weights

- **How To**: Hold a water bottle or use light weights in each hand. Perform movements such as lateral raises, front raises, and arm rotations.

- **Cardio Integration**: Integrate these movements with walking in place to keep the heart active.

- **Duration**: Combine 5-10 minutes of arm exercises with walking.

5. Brisk walk on a treadmill (if available)

- **How To**: Walk on a treadmill at a moderate pace.

- **Points of Caution**: Gradually increase speed and incline for greater intensity.

- **Duration**: 15-20 minutes, adapting to tolerance and ability.

6. Dynamic Stretching Combined with Movement

- **How to Do It**: Perform stretching movements such as lateral tilts or torso rotations, combining them with steps or marching in place.

- **Benefits**: This movement increases circulation and keeps the heart active.

- **Duration**: 10 minutes as part of the warm-up or cool-down.

Important Memories

- **Monitor Intensity**: Use conversation as a measure; the intensity is adequate if you can talk while exercising.

- **Listen to Your Body**: Any sign of pain or excessive fatigue indicates slowing down or stopping.

- **Regularity**: Maintaining a routine is essential to seeing continued progress.

By integrating these new cardio activities, Seniors over 60 can continue to improve their cardiovascular health, increase their endurance, and maintain a high overall well-being.

7. **Gentle and Rehabilitative Gymnastics**

Gentle gymnastics exercises for mobility and coordination

Gentle gymnastics is ideal for seniors over 60, combining light and controlled movements that help improve mobility and coordination. Here is a series of exercises focused on these aspects:

1. Arm rotations

- **How to Do It**: Sitting or standing, extend your arms to the side. Rotate your arms in small circles, first forward and then backward.

- **Benefits**: Improves shoulder mobility and warms up arm muscles.

- **Duration**: 2-3 minutes in each direction.

2. Lateral bends of the body

- **How to Do It**: Stand or sit, keep your back straight, and slowly lean your torso to one side and the other.

- **Benefits**: Increases lateral flexibility of the spine and strengthens the oblique muscles.

- **Repetitions**: 10-15 per side.

3. Knee raises

- **How to Do It**: When sitting in a chair, lift one knee towards your chest, lower it, and repeat with the other knee.

- **Benefits**: Improves hip mobility and strengthens lower abdominal muscles.

- **Repetitions**: 10-15 per leg.

4. Neck Rotations

- **How to Do It**: Sitting with your back straight, slowly turn your head from side to side, then tilt it forward and back.

- **Benefits**: Relieves tension in the neck and improves cervical flexibility.

- **Duration**: 2-3 minutes, performing the movement slowly.

5. Calf Stretch

- **How to Do It**: Standing near a wall for support, place one foot in front of the other and bend your front knee slightly, keeping your back heel on the ground.

- **Benefits**: Stretches the calves and improves the flexibility of the ankles.

- **Duration**: Maintain the stretch for 20-30 seconds per leg.

6. Balance Exercises on One Leg

- **How to Do It**: Stand up, lift one foot off the ground, and maintain balance for as long as possible. If necessary, use a chair or wall for support.

- **Benefits**: Improves balance and strengthens stabilizing muscles.

- **Duration**: Hold the position for 10-20 seconds per leg, gradually increasing the time.

7. Circular Movements of the Ankles

- **How to do it**: Sitting, extend one leg, and rotate the ankle first clockwise and then counterclockwise.

- **Benefits**: Improves ankle mobility and prevents stiffness.

- **Repetitions**: 10 rotations in each direction for each ankle.

Performance Tips

- **Controlled Movements**: Perform each movement in a slow and controlled manner to avoid injury.

- **Regularity**: Practice these exercises regularly for best results.

- **Listen to Your Body**: If an exercise causes pain or discomfort, it is essential to stop and, if necessary, consult a professional.

These gentle gymnastics exercises are specifically designed to improve the mobility and coordination of Seniors over 60, helping them maintain a high quality of life and excellent physical health.

Muscle relaxation techniques

Muscle relaxation techniques are essential for Seniors over 60 to reduce stress, relieve muscle tension, and improve overall well-being. Here are some detailed techniques:

1. Deep breathing

- **How to do it**: Sit comfortably or lie down, close your eyes, and focus on breathing. Inhale slowly through your nose, making your abdomen swell, and then exhale slowly through your mouth.

- **Duration**: Practice for 5-10 minutes.

- **Benefits**: Reduces stress and calms the mind, helping to relax muscles.

2. Progressive Muscle Relaxation

- **How to do it**: Lie down or sit comfortably. Tense a muscle group (such as your hands or feet) for a few seconds and then relax completely. Proceed progressively along the entire body.

- **Duration**: Approximately 20-30 minutes to go through all muscle groups.

- **Benefits**: Helps identify and reduce tension in specific muscle groups.

3. Gentle Stretching

- **How to Do It**: Light stretching exercises, such as slowly leaning forward from the seat or gently rotating your neck.

- **Duration**: 5-10 minutes.

- **Benefits**: Improves flexibility and reduces muscle stiffness.

4. Guided View

- **How to do it**: Sit or lie comfortably, close your eyes, and imagine relaxing scenarios, such as a quiet beach or a serene garden.

- **Duration**: 10-15 minutes.

- **Benefits**: Reduces stress and promotes inner peace, helping to relax the body.

5. Listening to Relaxing Music

- **How to**: Listen to calm music or nature sounds in a quiet environment.

- **Duration**: As desired, also during other relaxation activities.

- **Benefits**: Music has a calming effect on the mind and can help reduce muscle tension.

6. Mindfulness and Meditation techniques

- **How to do it**: Sit comfortably with your back straight, focus on the present, and observe your thoughts without judgment.

- **Duration**: 10-20 minutes per day.

- **Benefits**: Improves awareness of the body and mind, reducing muscle tension and stress.

7. Hot Bath

- **How to do it**: Take a warm bath, possibly adding bath salts or essential oils.

- **Duration**: 15-20 minutes.

- **Benefits**: Warm water helps relax muscles and relieves tension.

Performance Tips

- **Regularity**: Practice these techniques regularly for best results.

- **Quiet Environment**: Perform in a calm environment without distractions.

- **Listen to Your Body**: Adapt each technique to your abilities and comfort level.

By incorporating these muscle relaxation techniques into their daily routine, Seniors over 60 can significantly improve their quality of life by reducing stress and muscle tension.

30 day gentle gymnastics program

The following program is designed to progressively increase the mobility and coordination of seniors over 60 through gentle gymnastics exercises to be performed daily at home.

Week 1: Introduction and Basics

- **Exercises** :

    - **Arm Rotations**: Sitting or standing, rotate extended arms in slow circles. Do ten rotations forward and ten backward.

- **Lateral Body Flexions**: Standing or sitting, gently tilt your torso to one side and then to the other. Repeat ten times on each side.

- **Neck Rotations**: Sitting with your back straight, turn your head slowly from side to side and then tilt forward and backward. Five rotations in each direction.

- **Duration**: 15 minutes a day.

Week 2: Increased Mobility

- **Additional Exercises** :

  - **Knee Raises**: Sitting in a chair, alternately lift your knees towards your chest. Ten raises per leg.

  - **Calf Stretch**: Stand against a wall and push one foot back, keeping the heel on the ground, to stretch the calf. Do this for 20-30 seconds per leg.

- **Duration**: 20 minutes per day.

Week 3: Balance and Coordination

- **Additional Exercises** :

  - **One-Leg Balance**: Standing near a chair for support, lift one foot off the ground and balance for 10 to 20 seconds, then switch legs.

- **Circular Ankle Movements**: Sitting, extend one leg and rotate the ankle ten times in each direction, then change legs.

- **Duration**: 25 minutes per day.

Week 4: Consolidation

- **Routine**: Combine all the previous weeks' exercises, increasing each exercise's duration.

- **Additional Exercise** :

  - **Lateral Walking**: Walk from one side of the room to the other in a controlled manner, also moving your arms. This exercise takes 2-3 minutes.

- **Duration**: 30 minutes per day.

Performance Tips

- **Controlled Movements**: Perform each movement in a slow and controlled manner to avoid injury.

- **Listen to Your Body**: If an exercise causes pain or discomfort, it's essential to stop.

- **Warm-up and Cool-down**: Begin and end each session with a light warm-up and cool-down, such as a light walk or gentle stretching.

This 30-day program helps seniors over 60 progressively improve their mobility and coordination. Upon completion, participants should feel more agile, balanced, and coordinated in their daily activities.

Specific rehabilitation exercises

Joint-specific exercises are essential for maintaining mobility and relieving knee, shoulder, ankle, and wrist discomfort. Here are some detailed exercises:

Knee exercises

- **Seated Leg Extensions**: Sitting in a chair, extend one leg straight before you, then slowly lower it. Repeat 10-15 times per leg.

- **Flexion /Extension**: Sitting or lying down, slowly bend the knee, bringing the heel towards the buttocks, then extend the leg. 10-15 repetitions.

Shoulder exercises

- **Shoulder Rotations**: Standing or sitting, rotate your shoulders in circular motions, first forward and then backward, for ten rotations in each direction.

- **Bent Arm Side Raises**: Using a lightweight water bottle, raise your arms to the side, keeping them slightly bent to shoulder height, then lower them. 10-15 repetitions.

Ankle exercises

- **Ankle Rotations**: Sitting with legs extended, rotate the ankle clockwise and then counterclockwise for ten rotations in each direction per ankle.

- **Flexion /Extension**: Sitting or lying, push your feet forward and then pull them towards you to stretch the front and back of the ankle. 10-15 reps per ankle.

Wrist exercises

- **Wrist Rotations**: Extend one arm before you and rotate your wrist slowly and then counterclockwise. Ten rotations in each direction per wrist.

- **Wrist Flexion /Extension**: Keeping your arm extended, bend your wrist down and then up. 10-15 repetitions per wrist.

Finger exercises

- **Finger Stretch**: Open your hands, spreading your fingers as wide as possible, then close into a slow fist. 10-15 repetitions.

- **Pinching Motions**: Touch each fingertip with your thumb, one at a time, to improve finger mobility.

Execution Tips

- **Slow and Controlled Movements**: Avoid rapid or sudden movements to prevent joint stress.

- **Listen to Your Body**: Stop exercising if you feel pain and consult a professional if it persists.

- **Regularity**: Perform these exercises regularly to achieve the best results in terms of joint mobility and reduction of discomfort.

By incorporating these exercises into their daily routine, Seniors over 60 can help keep their joints flexible and functional, reducing the risk of stiffness and pain.

Post-30 Day Progression: Advanced Exercises

After completing the 30-day gentle exercise program, Seniors over 60 can move on to slightly more advanced exercises to continue improving their mobility, strength, and coordination. Here are a series of advanced exercises to incorporate into their daily routine:

1. Chair Squats

- **How to do it**: Place a chair behind you and pretend to sit, but without touching the chair, then stand up. Keep your back straight and bend your knees.

- **Benefits**: Strengthens legs and core, improving balance.

- **Repetitions**: 10-15 squats.

2. Lateral Leg Raises

- **How to do it**: Standing, with the support of a chair, lift one leg to the side, keeping it straight, then lower it. Alternate legs.

- **Benefits**: Improves lateral leg strength and balance.

- **Repetitions**: 10 per leg.

3. Sweet forward bends

- **How to do it**: Stand, slowly bend forward from the pelvis, trying to keep your legs straight. Extend your arms towards the floor and slowly return to standing.

- **Benefits**: Increases flexibility of the spine and legs.

- **Repetitions**: 8-10 push-ups.

4. Exercise "Bird Dog"

- **How to do it**: Extend one arm and the opposite leg simultaneously on all fours, maintaining balance. Return to the starting position and repeat with the other side.

- **Benefits**: Improves core control and balance.

- **Repetitions**: 10 per side.

5. Trunk Rotations

- **How to do it**: Sit in a chair and cross your arms over your chest. Rotate your torso from side to side without moving your hips.

- **Benefits**: Improves spinal mobility and torso flexibility.

- **Repetitions**: 10-15 per side.

6. Exercise "Dead Bug"

- **How to Do It**: Lying on your back, raise your bent knees and arms towards the ceiling. Alternatively, lower one arm and the opposite leg towards the floor without touching it.

- **Benefits**: Strengthens the core and improves coordination.

- **Repetitions**: 10 per side.

7. Combined Dynamic Stretching

- **How to Do It**: Combine stretching movements with balance elements, such as raising one leg and leaning sideways.

- **Benefits**: Improves flexibility and dynamic balance.

- **Duration**: 10-15 minutes.

Considerations for Execution

- **Gradual Increase**: Gradually increase the intensity and complexity of exercises.

- **Listen to Your Body**: Pay attention to how you feel while performing the exercises and reduce the intensity or stop if necessary.

- **Regularity**: Maintain a routine for best results.

These advanced exercises are designed to provide a more significant challenge than the initial 30-day program, helping Seniors over 60 improve their strength, mobility, and coordination safely and effectively.

8. Safety and Accident Prevention

Heating Techniques

Warming up prepares your body for physical activity by increasing blood flow to your muscles and reducing the risk of injury.

- **Light Walk or March in Place**: Begin with a light walk or march in place for 5-10 minutes. This helps to elevate your heart rate gradually.

- **Joint Rotations**: Includes rotations of the ankles, knees, hips, wrists, shoulders, and neck. Perform slow, controlled rotations in both directions for each joint.

- **Dynamic Stretching**: Exercises like leg swings (leg swings) and arm circles (arm rotations) involve fluid and controlled movements to prepare muscles and joints for exercise.

Cool-down techniques

Cooling down helps reduce muscle stiffness and recover after physical activity.

- **Gradual Cool-down**: Gradually reduce the intensity of physical activity, for example, from light jogging to walking, over 5-10 minutes.

- **Static Stretching**: After cooling down, perform static stretching, holding each position for 20-30 seconds. Focus on key muscle groups such as the calves, quadriceps, hamstrings, glutes, and lower back.

- **Deep Breathing**: Incorporate deep breathing exercises to relax your body and calm your heart rate. Inhale deeply through your nose and exhale slowly through your mouth.

Importance of Warm-up and Cool-down Techniques

- **Injury Prevention**: Warming up prepares muscles and joints for physical activity, reducing the risk of muscle strains or strains. Cooling down helps remove metabolic waste from muscles, preventing stiffness and pain.

- **Performance Improvement**: A good warm-up increases muscle efficiency, improving physical performance.

- **Cardiovascular Health**: Gradually increasing and decreasing exercise intensity protects the heart and circulatory system, especially in seniors over 60.

Adopting appropriate warm-up and cool-down techniques is crucial to safety and injury prevention. These practices should be an integral part of every exercise session for Seniors, helping to maintain their physical well-being and maximize the benefits of physical activity.

Warm-up and cool-down techniques

Warming up is fundamental before any physical exercise, especially for seniors. It prepares the body for activity, increasing muscle temperature and blood circulation and reducing the risk of injury.

Walk or March on the spot

- **How to do it**: Start with a slow walk or march in place, gradually increasing the intensity.

- **Duration**: Approximately 5-10 minutes.

- **Benefits**: Increases heart rate and warms muscles.

Joint Rotations

- **How To**: Perform slow, controlled rotations for your ankles, knees, hips, wrists, shoulders, and neck.

- **Duration**: Approximately 1 minute for each joint.

- **Benefits**: Improves joint mobility and reduces stiffness.

Dynamic Stretching

- **How to Do it**: Stretching involves fluid movements such as swings of the arms and legs, lateral inclinations of the body, and torso rotations.

- **Duration**: 5-10 minutes.

- **Benefits**: Prepares muscles and joints for physical activity.

Cool-down techniques

Cooling down helps the body return to a resting state after exercise. Normalizing circulation, reducing physical stress levels, and preventing muscle stiffness are essential.

Gradual Cooling

- **How to do it**: Reduce the intensity of physical activity, moving from vigorous to light walking or slow walking.

- **Duration**: 5-10 minutes.

- **Benefits**: Helps gradually reduce heart rate and blood pressure.

Static Stretching

- **How to Do It**: Perform slow, controlled stretches, holding each position for approximately 20-30 seconds. Focus on key muscle groups such as calves, quadriceps, hamstrings, glutes, and back.

- **Duration**: 10-15 minutes.

- **Benefits**: Reduces muscle tension and increases flexibility.

Deep breathing

- **How to do it**: Sitting or standing, practice deep breathing. Inhale through your nose, expand your abdomen, and exhale slowly through your mouth.

- **Duration** : 3-5 minutes.

- **Benefits**: Calms the nervous system and relaxes the body.

Proper warm-up and cool-down techniques are essential to safe and effective exercise, especially for seniors. These techniques help prevent injuries, improve performance, and promote rapid post-exercise recovery. Integrating them into your training routine improves exercise experience and overall well-being.

Accident prevention strategies

Injury prevention is crucial for Seniors, as injuries can have more severe impacts and longer recovery times. Here are some key strategies:

1. Muscle Strengthening and Balance Exercises

- **Description**: Incorporate exercises that increase muscle strength, particularly around critical joints such as the knees and hips, and that improve balance.

- **Execution**: Use light squats, leg raises, and yoga or tai chi.

- **Benefits**: Reduces the risk of falls and injuries related to instability.

2. Adequate warm-up and cool-down

- **Description**: Begin each exercise session with a warm-up and conclude with a cool-down.

- **Execution**: Light walking, dynamic stretching for warm-up, static stretching, and deep breathing to cool down.

- **Benefits**: Prevents muscle tears and helps reduce the accumulation of lactic acid.

3. Maintain Adequate Hydration

- **Description**: Drink sufficient water before, during, and after exercise.

- **Execution**: Always carry a bottle of water and drink regularly.

- **Benefits**: Prevents dehydration and muscle cramps.

4. Wear Appropriate Shoes and Clothing

- **Description**: Use shoes with good support and cushioning and comfortable clothing.

- **Execution**: Choose activity-specific shoes and clothing that do not restrict movement.

- **Benefits**: Reduces the risk of falls and injuries related to slipping or movement limitations.

5. Adapt the Exercises to Your Abilities

- **Description**: Modify the exercises to suit your fitness level and pre-existing conditions.

- **Execution**: Consult a fitness instructor or physical therapist for customized adjustments.

- **Benefits**: Prevents injuries related to overload and improper movements.

6. Avoid Overloading

- **Description**: Avoid increasing the intensity or duration of exercises too quickly.

- **Execution**: Gradually increase the intensity and listen to your body's signals.

- **Benefits**: Prevents overuse injuries such as tendonitis or muscle tears.

7. Regular check-ups and medical visits

- **Description**: Perform regular checkups to monitor your overall health and physical condition.

- **Execution**: Periodic visits to the doctor and, if necessary, to specialists such as physiotherapists.

- **Benefits**: Early identification of potential health problems that could increase the risk of injury.

8. Balanced nutrition

- **Description**: Maintain a balanced diet to support physical activity.

- **Execution**: Consume a diet rich in fruits, vegetables, lean proteins, and complex carbohydrates.

- **Benefits**: It provides the energy needed for exercise and helps with muscle regeneration.

By implementing these strategies, Seniors over 60 can significantly reduce their risk of injury. Maintaining an active and safe lifestyle is crucial to overall health and well-being at this age.

Pain management and injury recovery

Pain management and injury recovery are crucial aspects of maintaining a high quality of life in seniors. Here are some essential strategies and techniques:

1. Adequate rest

- **Importance**: Giving the body time to rest and heal is essential after an injury.

- **Execution**: Avoid activities that strain the injured part and ensure you get quality sleep.

- **Benefits**: Prevents further damage and speeds up the healing process.

2. Use of Cold and Heat

- **Cold Technique**: Apply ice packs to the injured area immediately after the injury to reduce swelling and pain.

- **Warm Technique**: Use warm compresses or warm baths in the later stages to relieve muscle stiffness.

- **Guide**: Alternate cold and heat, according to the instructions of your doctor or physiotherapist.

3. Physiotherapy and Rehabilitation Exercises

- **Description**: Follow a physical therapy program to restore strength, mobility, and function.

- **Execution**: Specific exercises under the guidance of a physiotherapist, starting gradually and increasing the intensity.

- **Benefits**: Helps you recover faster and prevent future injuries.

4. Pain Management

- **Medications**: Use painkillers prescribed by your doctor if necessary.

- **Alternative Techniques**: To manage pain, practice relaxation techniques such as deep breathing, meditation, or yoga.

- **Consultation**: Always consult a doctor before starting any pain management regimen.

5. Adequate Nutrition

- **Diet**: Consume foods rich in nutrients that promote healing, such as protein, vitamin C, and calcium.

- **Hydration**: Drink plenty of water to help your body heal.

6. Gradual Activities

- **Resumption of Activity**: Slowly begin to reintroduce physical activity, following the advice of your physical therapist or doctor.

- **Low-Impact Exercises: Start with low-impact** activities such as walking or swimming, avoiding strain on the injured part.

7. Listen to your body

- **Self-Observation**: Be aware of how your body feels during and after physical activity.

- **Warning Signs**: Pay attention to any signs of pain or discomfort and stop if necessary.

Managing pain and recovering from injuries takes time, patience, and adjusting your daily habits. By following these strategies, Seniors can improve their chances of a full recovery and reduce the risk of future injuries. It is essential to consult healthcare professionals for personalized advice and an appropriate recovery plan.

9. Post-30 Day Maintenance and Growth

Creating a long-term training regimen

Developing a long-term exercise regimen helps Seniors over 60 maintain health, mobility, and independence. Here's how to create a compelling and sustainable program:

1. Definition of Objectives

- **Set Realistic Goals**: Set clear, achievable goals, such as improving strength, balance, or flexibility.

- **Personalization**: Adjust goals based on your health, preferences, and fitness level.

2. Variation of Exercises

- **Diversification**: Combine different types of physical activity, such as walking, swimming, yoga, and gentle exercise, to work on different aspects of fitness.

- **Frequency**: Program different types of exercises during the week to prevent boredom and stimulate different muscle groups.

3. Gradual Increase

- **Progression**: Slowly increase the intensity and duration of exercises over time, avoiding abrupt changes.

- **Adjustments**: Make changes to your regimen based on your body's progress and feedback.

4. Monitoring and Evaluation

- **Progress Tracking**: Track exercises performed, intensity levels, and progress.

- **Periodic Evaluation**: Periodically review the program to evaluate its effectiveness and make any changes.

5. Integration of Physical Activity into Daily Life

- **Daily Activities**: Incorporate physical activity into daily activities, such as using the stairs instead of the elevator or gardening.

- **Consistency**: Maintain a consistent level of physical activity every day.

6. Prevention of Accidents

- **Warm-up and Cool-down**: Always include a warm-up before and a cool-down after exercise.

- **Safety Techniques**: Use appropriate equipment and follow correct techniques to reduce the risk of injury.

7. Listening to Your Body

- **Physical Response**: Pay attention to body signals, such as pain or excessive fatigue, and adjust your training accordingly.

- **Rest**: Make sure you have rest days to allow your body to recover.

8. Professional Support

- **Counseling**: Consider working with a personal coach or physical therapist to set up a suitable program, especially in the early stages.

9. Motivation and Social Involvement

- **Exercise Groups**: Join exercise groups or classes to increase motivation and enjoy the social aspect of physical activity.

- **Establish Routines**: Create regular habits to make exercise a natural part of your day.

A well-structured long-term training regime for Seniors over 60 is essential to promote overall health and well-being. The key is personalization, gradual progression, and listening to your body, ensuring that training is practical but also enjoyable and sustainable over time.

Introduction of new activities and challenges

To maintain a stimulating and beneficial long-term training regime, seniors over 60 need to introduce new activities and challenges periodically. This prevents monotony and helps improve various aspects of physical and mental health.

1. Exploring New Sports Disciplines

- **Activities**: Try age-appropriate sports like golf, pétanque or table tennis.

- **Benefits**: Improves coordination, strength, and social interaction.

2. Participation in Group Classes

- **Activities**: Join group classes such as water aerobics, dance, tai chi, or yoga.

- **Benefits**: Offers variety, socialization, and professional instruction.

3. Introduction of Outdoor Activities

- **Activities**: Include nature walks, hiking on easy trails, or gardening.

- **Benefits**: Increases vitamin D, improves mood, and offers movement diversity.

4. Short-Term Fitness Challenges

- **Activities**: Set small challenges, such as walking a certain distance or performing a specific number of repetitions of an exercise.

- **Benefits**: Motivates and provides a sense of accomplishment.

5. Use of Technology and Apps

- **Activities**: Use fitness apps with guided exercises, progress tracking, and virtual challenges.

- **Benefits**: Makes training interactive and easy to monitor.

6. Balance and Agility Exercises

- **Activities**: Add exercises that challenge balance and agility, such as the "stand on one foot" exercise or using a balance table.

- **Benefits**: Reduces the risk of falls and improves coordination.

7. Creative and Fun Activities

- **Activities**: Try activities like dance classes, tai chi, or yoga in unusual places (parks, beaches).

- **Benefits**: Increases interest and personal satisfaction.

8. Involvement in Community Events

- **Activities**: Participate in local events such as charity walks, walking groups, or activities organized by the community center.

- **Benefits**: Increases motivation through participation and community support.

Tips for Introducing New Businesses

- **Listen to Your Body**: Choose activities suited to your fitness level and state of health.

- **Consult Experts**: Talk to doctors or sports coaches before starting new challenging activities.

- **Maintain Safety**: Make sure new activities are safe and feasible.

Introducing new activities and challenges into the training regime of Seniors over 60 is a great way to keep training interesting and challenging. **This improves physical health and contributes to mental and social well-being.**

Tips for continuous improvement

To continuously improve fitness and overall health, Seniors over 60 need to adopt strategies that go beyond the essential advice already discussed. Here are some key aspects:

1. Progressive Adaptation of Intensity

- **Approach**: Gradually increase the intensity of exercises, rather than the duration, to improve endurance and strength without excessive fatigue.

- **Execution**: Add small weights to gentle gymnastics exercises or increase the intensity range in cardio exercises.

2. Exploration of New Forms of Movement

- **Tip**: Try activities outside of your regular fitness routine, such as exotic dancing, light water sports, or alternative forms of yoga.

- **Benefits**: Stimulates different muscle groups and mindsets, keeping training fresh and exciting.

3. Use of Innovative Technologies

- **Ideas**: Experiment with modern fitness equipment such as home pedal machines, advanced resistance bands, or virtual reality apps for exercise.

- **Benefits**: It keeps training stimulating and allows you to monitor your progress more precisely.

4. Integration of Mental Agility Activities

- **Examples**: Exercises that require coordination and strategic thinking, such as games of skill or sports that require planning and tactics.

- **Benefits**: Improves cognitive health and brain function along with physical fitness.

5. Wellbeing Self-Management Activities

- **Tips**: Practice self-massage techniques or learn the basics of pain self-management through methods such as acupressure.

- **Benefits**: Provides tools to manage muscle tension and discomfort independently.

6. Participation in workshops or seminars

- **Opportunities**: Join seminars or workshops on senior nutrition, stress management, or age-specific training techniques.

- **Benefits**: Provides additional knowledge and insights that can be integrated into your training routine.

7. Creation of a Support Community

- **How to**: Form a support group with friends or peers to share experiences, successes, and challenges.

- **Benefits**: Offers mutual motivation and a sense of belonging.

By adopting these insights and advanced strategies, Seniors over 60 can keep their fitness journey dynamic, challenging, and constantly evolving. The goal is to embrace a holistic approach to health and well-being, which considers the physical, mental, social, and cognitive aspects.

10. Conclusions

Final reflections

As we approach the conclusion of this journey dedicated to Seniors over 60, it is essential to reflect on the key aspects we have explored and how these can positively influence daily life and general well-being.

Appreciation of Your Body

- **Reflection**: Recognize and appreciate your body's resilience and capacity. Every step and every movement is a testimony to strength and determination.

- **Implication**: A positive attitude towards your body increases motivation and self-esteem.

Importance of Regular Physical Activity

- **Reflection**: Physical activity goes beyond simply maintaining physical fitness; it is a source of joy, a way to connect with others, and a powerful tool for maintaining independence.

- **Implication**: Integrate exercise into your daily routine as a rewarding habit.

Value of Socialization and Community Support

- **Reflection**: Social interactions and community support are crucial in improving quality of life and maintaining a positive mindset.

- **Implication**: Actively seek opportunities to socialize and build a support network.

Continuous Learning and Adaptation

- **Reflection**: Learning is a continuous process. Adapting exercise routines and adopting new wellness strategies is essential to addressing the challenges that accompany aging.

- **Implication**: Be open to change and willing to try new activities.

Prevention and Proactive Health Management

- **Reflection**: Prevention is vital to a long, healthy, active life. Proactively managing your health can make a big difference in preventing and mitigating various age-related conditions.

- **Implication**: Take a holistic approach to health, including exercise, nutrition, rest and stress management.

Gratitude and Positivity

- **Reflection**: Maintaining an attitude of gratitude and positivity can significantly influence your mental and physical well-being.

- **Implication**: Practice daily gratitude and look for the silver lining.

This journey through different facets of wellness for Seniors over 60 highlights the importance of a balanced and integrated approach to health and fitness. The ultimate goal is to live a whole, satisfying, and independent life, embracing each day with energy, determination, and a sense of fulfillment.

Motivation and inspiration to continue

In conclusion, it is essential to recognize the importance of motivation and inspiration in the fitness and well-being journey, especially for Seniors over 60. Reflecting on the wisdom that " ***Time passes for everyone, you can decide whether to use it to improve yourself or suffer it inexorably,*** " we can draw strength and determination to continue our journey.

Choose to Improve

- **Reflection**: Time is a precious and inevitable resource. The decision to use it to improve yourself is a powerful act of self-determination.

- **Implication**: Every day provides an opportunity to grow, learn and improve. Actively using the time to your advantage is a step towards a richer and more satisfying life.

Celebrate Small Successes

- **Strategy**: Recognize and celebrate every small milestone you reach, whether it's an increase in physical activity, a new exercise you learned, or a day when you felt perfect.

- **Benefits**: This recognition strengthens motivation and builds a sense of continuous progress.

Searching for Sources of Inspiration

- **Tip**: Find inspiring and motivating stories, people, or communities. This may include Senior athletes, exercise groups, or personal success stories.

- **Benefits**: Success stories can be powerful motivators and a reminder that meaningful goals can be achieved at any age.

Set New Goals

- **Approach**: After reaching a goal, set a new one. This can be related to exercise, socializing, learning, or personal well-being.

- **Benefits**: Keeps the mind and body engaged and constantly evolving.

Maintain a Positive Attitude

- **Importance**: Your attitude each day can make a big difference. Maintaining a positive approach helps you overcome challenges and see growth opportunities.

- **Strategy**: Practice optimism and resilience, celebrate your strengths, and gracefully accept the aspects of life that cannot be changed.

The decision to use time to improve yourself is a powerful way to live a whole and meaningful life. This choice leads to a sense of control and personal satisfaction, continually inspiring you to push yourself beyond your limits and thoroughly enjoy every moment. We remember that every day is a new opportunity to grow, learn, and flourish.

Giuseppe Di Mauro